YOUR KNOWLEDGE HAS VALUE

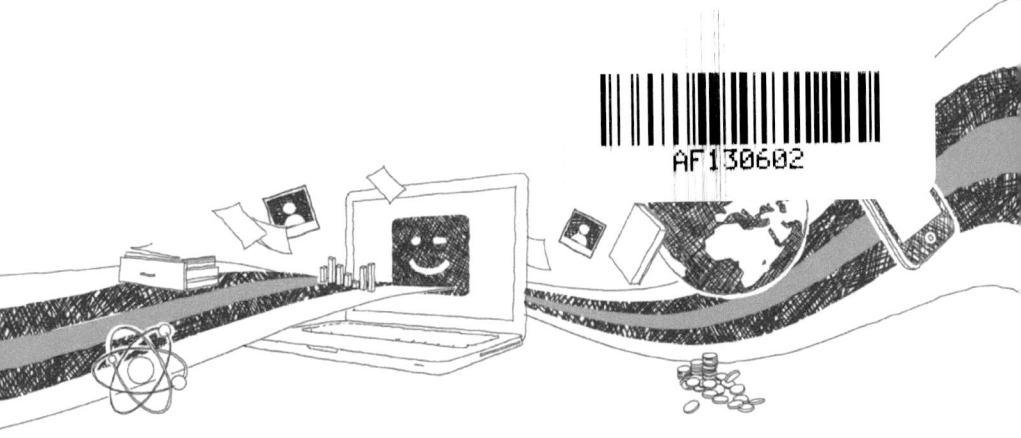

AF130602

- We will publish your bachelor's and master's thesis, essays and papers

- Your own eBook and book - sold worldwide in all relevant shops

- Earn money with each sale

Upload your text at www.GRIN.com and publish for free

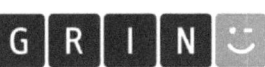

Bibliographic information published by the German National Library:

The German National Library lists this publication in the National Bibliography; detailed bibliographic data are available on the Internet at http://dnb.dnb.de .

Imprint:

Copyright © 2020 GRIN Verlag
Print and binding: Books on Demand GmbH, Norderstedt Germany
ISBN: 9783346179074

This book at GRIN:

https://www.grin.com/document/593460

Veena Soni

Food Security in India. Issues and Suggestions for Effectiveness

GRIN Verlag

GRIN - Your knowledge has value

Since its foundation in 1998, GRIN has specialized in publishing academic texts by students, college teachers and other academics as e-book and printed book. The website www.grin.com is an ideal platform for presenting term papers, final papers, scientific essays, dissertations and specialist books.

Visit us on the internet:

http://www.grin.com/

http://www.facebook.com/grincom

http://www.twitter.com/grin_com

FOOD SECURITY IN INDIA: ISSUES
AND
SUGGESTIONS FOR EFFECTIVENESs

INTRODUCTION

Attaining food security is a matter of prime importance for India where more than a-third of its population is estimated to be absolutely poor, and as many as one half of its children have suffered from malnourishment over the last three decades. Several important issues have emerged in the context of food security in India. These have been (a) the liberalization of the economy and its impact on agriculture and food security; (b) the establishment of the WTO and the agreement on Agriculture; (c) climate change and its impact on food production and prices; (d) the prevalence of hunger and poverty coexisting with high levels of food stocks; (e) the introduction of the targeted Public Distribution System (f) the „Right to Food" campaign; and (g) the National Food Security Bill. These important issues have posed severe challenges for food security in the country.

The Food and Agricultural Organization (FAO) states that food security emerges when all people at all times have physical and economic access to sufficient, safe and nutritious food to meet their dietary needs and food preferences for an active and healthy life. Food security has three important and closely related components, which are availability of food, access to food, and absorption of food.

Food security is thus a multi-dimensional concept and extends beyond the production availability, and demand for food. There has been a definite and significant paradigm shift in the concept of food security from mere macro level availability and stability to micro level household food insecurity, and also from an assessment of energy intake to measures and indicators of malnutrition.

1. FOOD SECURITY IN INDIA: A BRIEF OVERVIEW

The green revolution initiated in the late 1960s was a historic watershed that transformed the food security situation in India. It tripled food grain production over the next three or four decades and consequently reduced by over 50 percent both the levels of food insecurity and poverty in the country, this was achieved in spite of the increase in population during the period, which almost doubled. The country succeeded in the laudable task of becoming a food self-sufficient nation, at least at the macro level.

The per capita dietary energy supply increased significantly from 2370 kcal/day in the early 1990s to about 2440 kcal/day in 2001-03 and to 2550 kcal/day in 2006-08. The prevalence of undernourishment in the total population also decreased from 25 to 20 per cent during the period of 1990 to 2000, and as many as 58 million individuals were estimated to have come out of the poverty trap. The absolute number of poor persons came down from 317 million to 259 million with other livelihood indicators such as the literacy rate and longevity increasing substantially. The life expectancy at birth for males and females respectively, in 2005-06 was 63 and 66 years respectively as compared to that in 1986-91, which was as low as 58 and 59 years for males and females respectively. (Agricultural Statistics at a Glance; 2007).

Table 1A: Per Capita Dietary Energy Supply and Prevalence of
Under Nutrition in Total Population.

Year	Dietary Energy Supply (Kcal/day)	Undernourishment in the Total Population (%)
1990-92	2370	25
1995-97	2450	21
2002-2004	2470	20
2006-2008*	2550	20

Source: FAO, RAP, 2007/15 and FAO Year Book 2012.

Notwithstanding the achievement of macro level food security and the discernable improvement in per capita consumption, the country is still home to a-fifth of the world"s undernourished population. This given situation has been ascribed to high and increasing population pressure with nearly 16 million people being added annually to the already large population exceeding 1.2 billion. This situation of hunger and malnutrition is also equally on account of serious problems related to the distribution and economic access to food, which adversely affect household and individual level food insecurities.

According to the FAO"s latest food security report, micronutrient and vitamin A deficiency were the prime determinants to child health and nutrition in India. It is reported that nearly 57 percent of pre-school children suffered from vitamin A deficiency, a significantly higher level as compared to even Sub Saharan Africa. The infant mortality rate in India (for infants under one year) was as high as 56 in 2005. The NFHS-3 reported that 19 percent of India"s children were wasted, 38 percent stunted, and 46 percent were underweight, figures that are disturbing and far from satisfactory.

The extent and nature of food insecurity can be broadly categorized into (1) Chronic Food Insecurity (2) Nutritional Insecurity (3) Food Insecurity caused by lack of Food Absorption, and (4) Transitory Food Insecurity. There are several factors, both on the supply side, as well as the demand side that may cause chronic food insecurity. The most important supply side determinants of food insecurity are (*a*) the level of domestic food production, (*b*) the imports of food and (*c*) the distribution of food (PDS). The determinants on the demand side are (*i*) the growth of population (*ii*) the purchasing power; (*iii*) product prices/subsidies and (*iv*) the extent and effectiveness of supportive social programmes and schemes such as the ICDS, the Mid Day Meal scheme, Food for Work Programmes, and Rural Wage Employment Programmes.

2. THE AVAILABILITY OF FOOD

National Food Security is critically dependent on the adequate availability of sufficient food stocks to fully satisfy domestic demand at all times. This requirement can be ensured either through domestic food production or through imports. We must therefore first have a close look at the performance in terms of food availability and also the policies pursued in order to ensure that sufficient food is available to meet domestic demand.

The Status and Trends in Food Production and Availability

National self-sufficiency in food grain has been a major achievement in post-Independence India. Having remained a severely food deficit economy over two decades after Independence, India managed to achieve self-sufficiency in food grain production at the macro or national level. The green revolution ushered in a dramatic and steady increase in domestic food grain production practically eliminating the need for food imports, except to a very limited extent in times of extreme emergencies such as droughts and serious crop failure. Food grain production in the country registered a steady increase over two decades from only 50 million tonnes in 1950-51 to 244.5 million tonnes in 2010-11. The growth rate in food grain has been about 2.5 percent per annum during the post Independence period. Moreover the production of oilseeds, sugarcane, fruits, vegetables and milk has also increased significantly.

A closer look at the experience in the last two decades however indicates a tapering off or decline in both production and yields. It has been observed (S. Mahendra Dev, and A. Sharma 2011) that during the period 1996-2008 as compared to the years 1986-97, the growth rate in food grain production declined very sharply from nearly 3 percent to around 0.93 percent. Moreover the growth in production was much less than the growth in population in the latter period, having a serious impact on per capita availability. The growth rate of yields in food grain also declined from 3.21 percent to 1.04 percent. There was thus a decline in rates of production and yields for cereals, pulses, oilseeds, rice and wheat as seen in Table 1B below.

These being fitted trend rates based on CACP, 2009.

Major Factors Responsible for Decline in Food Production

The performance in the agriculture sector is extremely vital for ensuring adequate availability and access to food; this is more so because more than 55 percent of the country"s population depends on this primary sector. The more recent status of the agriculture sector and the factors primarily responsible for the disturbing slowdown in this sector provide a clear explanation for the notable decline in the growth of food production.

Agricultural growth in the country was quite high from the Fifth Plan to the Ninth Plan and reached its peak of 5.7 percent during the Sixth Plan period. It has however declined significantly during the Tenth and Eleventh Plan. Over a longer period we see that the growth rate has declined from 3.5 percent per annum from 1981-92 to 1996-97, to about 2.0 percent or even lower from

1997-98 to 2004-05. However, there have been some encouraging signs of improvement in recent years.

Table 1B: Growth Rate and Yields of Food grain, Oilseeds and Pulses
(percent per annum)

Crop Group/crops	Production		Yields	
	1986-87 to 1996-97	1996-97 to 2007-08	1986-87 to 1996-97	1996-97 to 2007-08
Food grains	2.93	0.93	3.21	1.04
Cereals	3.06	0.97	3.36	1.19
Coarse cereals	1.19	1.53	3.66	2.25
Pulses	1.32	0.36	1.49	-0.02
Oilseeds	6.72	1.99	3.32	1.49
Rice	3.06	1.02	2.37	1.22
Wheat	4.09	0.65	2.93	0.34

Source: *As in S.Mahendra Dev, and A. Sharma, 2011. There being filled trend rates based on CACP, 2009.*

Indian agriculture faces both short run and long run constraints and problems. These are reflected in widespread farmers suicides which are increasing in some states. With declining growth in yields, farming is increasingly becoming a non-viable activity. With rising land degradation, loss of soil fertility and water logging, the problems faced by the farming community are on the rise. The fall in ground water levels and decline in surface irrigation are being faced in several regions.

The significant differences in productivity across regions and among different crops, as also between irrigated and non-irrigated farmland is giving rise to regional disparities and resulting inequalities. These domestic constraints accompanied by our exposure to international competition and international price volatility has affected domestic agriculture progressively in the recent past. The shrinking of farm size due to sub division and land alienation is aggravating the agrarian crisis. The diversion of agricultural land to set up special economic zones, the change in land use due to urbanization and the alienation of tribal land for mining and other industrial activities are other important issues that pose severe challenges to the farming community.

There are several other important reasons that have emerged as factors responsible for the deceleration of agricultural growth since the mid 90s (GoI 2007). Most important among them is the slowing down of public and private investment in agriculture and rural infrastructure. There has been a marked decline in investment related to irrigation, technological change and diversification of agriculture, and fertilizer use in spite of a significant increase in agricultural credit. However, there is some evidence related to the revival of agricultural growth in recent years but this trend is far from encouraging keeping in mind the vital role of the agricultural sector in ensuring food security and livelihoods.

Per Capita Availability of Food Grains

At the macro level the availability of food grain is calculated as 87.5 percent of the gross production (with the rest accounting for seeds, farm animal feed and waste) plus imports minus the changes in stocks held by the government. Assuming no net change in private stocks this can be treated as representing the overall food grain consumption in the country.

The pre-independence period witnessed a rapid decline in per capita availability of food grains from about 545 gm per day to a level as low as 407 gm per day. This was largely on account of the policies of the colonial government. However on the basis of five year averages India witnessed a significant rise in net availability from a level of 416 gm per day in 1950-55 to a level of 485 gm per day during the period 1989-91 (Patnaik, 2004). However since the early 1990s there has been a significant fall in food grain availability to a level of 445 gm per day by the year 2006-07 (Saxena N.C., 2011).

The per capita net availability is estimated to have increased by a mere 10 percent over a 56-year period from 1951 to 2007. However, the net availability of food grain has declined if one compares the level of 469 gm per day in 1960 with a mere 443 gm per day as reported in the year 2007. This implies that significant increases in food grain production have not been able to keep up with the increase in population. It is important to mention here that there has been a steady decline in net per capita food grain availability in the post-economic reforms period of 1991 to 2007, with the levels falling from 501 gm per day in 1991 to only 443 gm per day in 2007.

According to some analysts, this was also on account of the export of nearly seven million tonnes of food grain per annum during the period 2002 to 2007. This export of food grain at highly subsidized prices to tackle the low world prices was preferred over undertaking widespread internal distribution of food grain to those in need (Saxena N.C., 2011). It may also be seen from Table 2 below that while net availability of cereals declined from a level of 468.5 gm per day in 1991 to a level of 407.4 gm per day in 2007, the net availability of pulses which is a major protein source in the Indian diet declined significantly during the same period. While it was 41.6 gm per day in 1991, it fell to a level as low as 31.5 gm per day in 2005 but improved significantly to 35.5 gm per day in the next two years though it is still below the stipulated norms.

On the other hand the per capita net availability of edible oils and sugar has increased over the years, more due to an increasing level of imports than on account of any impressive increase in domestic oilseed production.

Table 2: Net Availability of Cereals, Pulses, Edible Oils, Vanaspati and Sugar

Year	Per Capita net availability per day (grams)			Edible Oil (Kg)	Vanaspati (Kg)	Sugar (Nov.-Oct.) (Kg.)
	Cereals	Pulses	Total Food grain			
1951	334.2	60.7	394.9	2.5*	0.7*	5.0*
1961	399.7	69.0	468.7	3.2	0.8	4.8
1971	417.6	51.2	468.8	3.5	1.0	7.4
1981	417.3	37.5	454.8	3.8	1.2	7.3
1990	435.3	41.1	476.4	5.3	1.1	12.3
1991	468.5	41.6	510.1	5.5	1.0	12.7
1992	434.5	34.3	468.8	5.4	1.0	13.0
1993	427.9	36.2	464.1	5.8	1.0	13.7
1994	434.0	37.2	471.2	6.1	1.0	12.5
1995	457.6	37.8	495.4	6.3	1.0	13.2
1996	442.5	32.7	475.2	7.0	1.0	14.1
1997	466.0	37.1	503.1	8.0	1.0	14.6
1998	414.2	32.8	447.0	6.2	1.0	14.5
1999	429.2	36.5	465.7	8.5	1.3	14.9
2000	422.7	31.8	454.4	9.0	1.4	15.6
2001	386.2	30.0	416.2	8.2	1.3	15.8
2002	458.1	35.4	494.1	8.8	1.4	16.0
2003	408.5	29.1	437.6	7.2	1.4	16.3
2004	426.9	35.8	462.7	9.9	1.2	16.8
2005	390.9	31.5	422.4	10.2	1.1	15.5
2006	412.8	32.5	445.3	10.6	1.1	16.3
2007	407.4	35.5	442.8	11.1	1.2	16.8
2008	394.2	41.8	436.0	11.4	1.2	17.8
2009	407.4	37.0	444.0	12.7	1.3	18.8
2010	401.7	35.4	437.1	13.3	1.1	17.9
2011(P)	423.5	39.4	462.9	13.6	1.0	17.0

Sources: *Economic Survey 2008-2009*, and 2012-13, Government of India.
Note: *Pertains to the year 1955-56

Changes in Consumption Patterns

Though there was a marked rise in per capita real expenditure from 1972-73 to 2004-05, the per capita cereal intake declined in both rural and urban areas. This fall in cereal consumption was however accompanied by an increase in the consumption of non-cereal food. It is clearly evident that in the post green revolution period there has been diversification in the food consumption patterns, and the share of cereal consumption in total household consumption has declined in rural and urban areas. In Table 3 these changes in the food basket are shown for different deciles of rural and urban population.

Table 3: Percentage of Cereal Consumption in Household Budget for different Income Groups in both Rural and Urban Sectors

Year	Rural				Urban			
	Bottom 30%	Middle 40%	Top 30%	All	Bottom 30%	Middle 40%	Top 30%	All
1970-71	53.65	43.65	29.49	38.15	38.85	28.19	13.37	21.58
1990-91	39.37	30.68	18.22	25.93	27.55	19.13	9.49	15.12
1993-94	35.68	27.87	15.72	22.95	25.59	17.14	8.18	13.32
2004-05	29.34	22.04	12.49	18.28	20.59	13.29	6.29	10.21

Source: *NSS Consumer Expenditure Surveys*, Government of India.
Note: The shares are derived from the expenditure at constant prices (1993-94 prices)

It is seen in Table 3 that the share of cereals in total consumption has declined notably even for the lowest three deciles of the population in both rural and urban areas. However, the fall in cereals consumption varies considerably for the different income groups with the middle and higher deciles accounting for a sharper reduction. This is an expected trend as income increases. However, the decline in cereal consumption by the three poorest deciles of the population in both rural and urban areas is a matter of concern as these groups meet a large proportion of their nutritional requirements through cereal consumption while their access to non-cereal foods is limited and is also affected by the different prices of cereal and non-cereals. This trend seems to strongly indicate a lowering of the energy requirements of the poor and has a serious nutritional implication that needs to be carefully examined.

Projected Supply and Demand for Food

Several studies have attempted to estimate the future demand and supply scenario for food in the country (Kumar, P., 1998; Bhalla, G.S. et al, 2001;Dyson, T. and Hanchate, A., 2000). Most of these studies have predicted a comfortable demand-supply balance for food grain during the coming decade. While India is expected to be self sufficient in food grains, it would have to continue importing pulses and oilseeds to meet its future requirements.

The projected demand and supply for the year 2020 has been estimated by the Ministry of Agriculture as seen in Table 4 below.

Table 4: Estimated Production and Projected Demand of Cereals and Non-Cereals

Crop	2008-09			2011-12			2020
	Projected Demand	Projected Production	Surplus/ shortfall	Projected Demand	Projected Production	Surplus/ shortfall	Projected Demand
Rice	92.87	99.15	6.28	98.79	104.21	5.42	111.9
Wheat	72.72	80.58	7.86	77.36	83.61	6.25	79.9
Coarse cereals	35.9	39.48	3.58	38.19	35.75	-2.44	37.3
Pulses	17.51	14.66	-2.85	19.91	15.73	-4.18	23.8
Food grains	219.0	233.88	14.88	234.26	239.3	5.04	252.8
Sugarcane	275.9	271.25	-4.66	322.54	305.51	-17.03	--
Oilseeds	47.4	28.16	-19.27	53.39	27.53	-25.86	--

Source: Ministry of Agriculture (2009)

The figures in Table 4 indicate that while the balance in food grain is expected to be maintained with enough supply to meet the projected demand in 2020, there is likely to be a shortfall in the case of coarse cereals, pulses, oilseeds as well as sugarcane. Thus the reliance on imports is likely to continue in pulses and oilseeds in particular till the year 2020.

Performance of the Food Management System

A nationwide public distribution system, which transfers available supplies to entitled consumers, is entirely run by the State Governments. It is closely supported by the Central Government through procurement of food grain from the surplus regions as well as by maintaining buffer stocks. This Central Government initiative intended to protect and incentivize farmers, is an effort to strengthen production and thereby self-sufficiency in food grains. The maintenance of buffer stocks by the Central Government on the other hand is intended to guard against volatility in basic food grain prices and achieve the necessary moderation in the prices of food grain in the open market in the event of any unforeseen fall in production, which takes place mainly due to climatic conditions such as drought. The buffer stock thus provides an effective means of intervention by the Centre in order to control prices and ensure availability and access to the especially vulnerable population.

The food management system and food price policy thus consists of three major instruments, namely procurement at minimum support prices, the maintenance of buffer stocks, and the public distribution system. As the procurement and buffer stocking activity falls largely within the ambit of the Central Government and has a critical impact on macro level availability and market prices of food grain, we will confine our discussion here to these two important food system interventions, and cover the PDS which ensures access to food grain and other essential commodities in the section regarding access and nutritional issues.

MSP and Procurement

While support price policy for agricultural commodities seeks to assure remunerative prices to farmers in order to ensure higher production and investment, it also tries to safeguard the interest of consumers by ensuring supplies at affordable and reasonable prices, through the provision of subsidy. It may be mentioned here that the benefits of the minimum support prices (MSP) offered to farmers depends on the level of awareness of farmers, which is still reported to be quite low (NSSO 59th Round 2003).

The MSP announced for each year is fixed by the State on the basis of recommendations of the CACP. During the last decade the MSP has increased sharply as compared to the earlier decade. The MSP for paddy of common variety increased by as much as nearly 70 percent during the short span of 2004-05 to 2009-10 as compared to a rise of only 9.8 percent for the period 2000-01 to 2004-05. Similarly there has been a sharp increase of MSP for wheat by 71.0 percent in the second half of the last decade as compared to the first half wherein the MSP for wheat grew at a mere 8.6 percent.

Table 5: Procurement of Rice and Wheat.

Year	Wheat	Rice
2003-04	15.8	22.8
2004-05	16.8	24.6
2005-06	14.8	27.7
2006-07	9.2	25.1
2007-08	11.1	28.7
2008-09	22.7	33.2
2009-10	25.3	32.0
2010-11	22.5	34.2
2011-12	28.3	35.0

Source: Department of Food and Public Distribution System, GoI, 2009, and *Economic Survey 2012-13*.

The growing concern for maintaining adequate stocks for effective price interventions in the event of unforeseen declines in production and resulting food insecurity seems to be the reason for the escalating MSP, and food grain procurement has certainly responded to this by increasing significantly in the recent years, as seen in Table 5.

Buffer Stocks

The maintenance of a buffer stock is important for ensuring national food security. Stocks mainly of rice and wheat are regularly maintained from year to year at a substantial cost in order to effectively take care of variations in domestic food grain output. These variations occur quite regularly due to climate and man-made factors. Buffer stocks are created from the domestic food surpluses available in years of high production. They are also built and maintained through imports as and when necessary. The optimum size of the buffer stocks at any point of time is based on the suggestions of expert committees appointed for the purpose by the government from time to time. At present the size of the buffer stock varies between 15 and 25 million tonnes according to seasonal requirements.

Table 6: Buffer Stock of Food grains (in million tonnes)

Year	1st July Actual Buffer Stock	1st July Norm of Buffer Stock
2002	63.0	24.3
2003	35.2	24.3
2004	29.9	24.3
2005	24.5	24.3
2006	19.4	24.3
2007	23.9	24.3
2008	36.2	24.3
2009	52.5	24.3

Source: Department of Food and Public Distribution System, GoI, 2009

The trend in buffer stocking over the last decade are indicated in Table 6. The figures show the actual level of buffer stocks available over the years as compared to the norm that has been stipulated.

The steep and perpetual rise in MSP, accompanied by the rise in issue prices combined with the obligation to mop up all the stocks offered by farmers led to a steep rise in the buffer stock to a level of 63 million tonnes in 2002 far exceeding the norms, of 25 million tonnes as on 1ˢᵗ July 2002.

The severe drought in 2003 led to a drawing down of the buffer stock in subsequent years and in 2006-07 the levels fell substantially below the norms. This forced the government to import wheat during the years 2006-07. With a spike in production and procurement in 2008 the level of buffer stocks again rose sharply to a level substantially higher than the norms. Buffer stocks exceeded the stipulated norm in 2008 and 2009, however this helped in effectively cushioning shortfalls caused by the drought in 2009. Droughts seem to occur with greater frequency mainly as a consequence of climate change and uncertain weather and perhaps it is time to seriously review the norms for buffer stocking though this would further increase the financial burden of the Central Government. De-centralization of both procurement and buffer stocking seems to be the only way out with the greater sharing of responsibilities between the Centre and the states in order to ensure food security and manage the food system in the days ahead.

Measures and Policies for Sustaining and Strengthening Availability

The health of the agricultural sector and its sustained growth and development is central to ensuring national level availability of cereal and non-cereal food. The major areas of concern for the sector are (*a*) infrastructure, (*b*) land and water management, (*c*) agricultural research and extension, (*d*) agricultural inputs and credit, (*e*) effective marketing and price policies, (*f*) diversification, and (*g*) development and strengthening of institutions to effectively meet the challenges posed by these concerns.

Infrastructure requires increasing investment, which is inversely related to the level of subsidies. The only way to increase investment in essential agricultural infrastructure is thus to reduce unsustainable subsidies. This would provide resources for public investment and larger outlays for infrastructure. Public investment is always seen to lead private investment, and both are crucial for enhancing agricultural growth. Though gross capital formation in agriculture has increased in recent years, it needs to go up substantially in order to enable the achievement of higher levels of agricultural growth as compared to the present level which is disturbingly low, and which has been declining steadily in recent years.

The second factor that has adversely affected the growth of productivity in the agricultural sector in recent times is the notable deterioration in soil quality, water shortages, as well as the rapid depletion in ground water. The sustenance of soil health and the management of water resources thus require immediate attention.

There is an urgent need to enhance water conservation measures and the efficient and sustainable use of water. Proper water management involving investments in irrigation, watershed development, and community based water conservation measures require a boost. The restructuring of fertilizer subsidies by making them nutrient based is a desirable move and is likely to lead to a more balanced use of fertilizers that will go a long way in improving soil quality.

The lack of proper knowledge and awareness among Indian farmers with regard to existing technologies is yet another important constraint that affects the performance of the agricultural sector. The only way to improve this situation is to strengthen the agricultural training of extension staff. With wide variations in the agro-climatic conditions in different regions in the country especially in backward agricultural areas, research efforts require to be location specific particularly focused on region specific resources, patterns and practices in farming. The pioneering work in this direction initiated by the M.S. Swaminathan Research Foundation has been commendable and should be widely extended to more regions.

Yet another important factor in the sustained growth of the agricultural sector is the flow and availability of farm credit. In spite of a small increase in the flow of farm credit there has hardly been any improvement in the credit for small and marginal farmers. The credit deposit rates especially of rural and semi-urban branches of banks have declined indicating a neglect of the credit needs of the farming community. There has also been an increase in indirect credit in total agricultural credit. This indirect credit has been through various intermediary agencies and instruments such as the R.E.C., special bonds issued by NABARD, and deposits placed by banks in the Rural Infrastructure Development Fund in lieu of priority sector lending (Saxena, N.C. 2011).

There have also been significant regional inequalities in the provisioning of credit with a professional reluctance by banks to operate in rural areas and particularly in remote and undeveloped agricultural regions. In these areas small and marginal farmers are being left to the mercy of private informal lenders and usurious moneylenders especially at a time when the monetization of agricultural inputs has been increasing sharply, causing high levels of indebtedness and distress.

There have also been a serious deficiency in proper and effective marketing institutions and arrangements, and as a result there are not only output price volatility but also and increasing un-bridged gap between producer and consumer prices with large margins being siphoned off by intermediaries.

Collective marketing through self help groups, small producer cooperatives and contract farming, and direct sales to corporate and urban chain stores needs to be encouraged and supported by the government in order to ensure the viability of small and marginal farmers in particular.

It is also observed that diversion of land into non-agricultural use has also shown an increasing trend. The need to set up Special Economic Zones to boost industrial production and exports also diverts agricultural land to non-agricultural use (Bhramanand, P.S.,et al. 2013). These trends would affect agricultural growth and food security if not strictly regulated. However with increases in yields and productivity there would be a possibility of putting land to non-agricultural usage. It is essential to evolve policies and criteria by which the most appropriate lands are identified for the purpose of non-agricultural use.

Increasing climate change is also likely to impact agriculture and so there are very valid reasons to be concerned regarding this phenomenon. Moreover a large segment of the population is dependent on sectors like agriculture, forestry and fishery, which are extremely sensitive to sudden and unforeseen changes in the climate. Climate change, which results in both increases and decreases in rainfall, rising temperature, and rising sea levels can bring about droughts and floods with increasing severity. This is bound to threaten food security and livelihoods in the country.

Recent policy initiatives such as the National Action Plan on climate change needs to be vigorously pursued, improved upon and effectively implemented as successful adaptation strategies and mitigation measures are most essential for sustainable long term agricultural development and food security.

In addition to the problems identified above there are other challenges facing Indian agriculture such as globalization and the resulting volatility in prices, the disturbing trends in rapidly declining farm sizes, and increasing environmental stress. There is thus a need for substantial increase in public outlays for agriculture, especially rural infrastructure while simultaneously improving and strengthening the delivery mechanisms. The relative neglect of the agricultural sector as compared to the industrial and service sectors must be avoided and the government must provide a big push to agriculture specially in order to ensure future food security and the planned expansion in the food system to be able to ensure its increasing rights based obligations.

3. THE STATE OF ACCESS TO FOOD AND NUTRITION (ABSORPTION)

For individuals food security means that they have access to the required food either through their own production, through the market, and through the governments transfer mechanism. Food security requires the poor to have adequate purchasing power apart from physical access to the required food. Very often the poor cannot afford to obtain the available food due to the high level of market prices, therefore, various social protection programmes are needed to ensure access. The sufficient purchasing power in the hands of the poor can be made available through an employment intensive pattern of growth wherein remunerative work is provided to the poor thereby enhancing their purchasing power. The other way of improving access is by increasing incomes and subsidizing food through social protection measures such as employment generation programmes and the provision of affordable and subsidized food through PDS.

Adequate availability and access to food does not necessarily mean that the food would be absorbed to ensure higher levels of nutrition. Food absorption by the human body is a major problem particularly in rural areas and urban slums. According to researchers the „capacity to be nourished (for the body to absorb food) depends crucially to other characteristics of a person that are influenced by non-food factors such as medical attention, health services, basic education, sanitary arrangements, provision of clean water, eradication of infectious epidemics and so on‟ (Dreze, J. and A. Sen, 1989). This inability to absorb the food intake or where the body is incapable of absorbing the nutrients from the food consumed can be termed absorption food insecurity.

The State of Access to Food

It is seen from NSS data that there has been a significant reduction in the level of hunger at the household level. The data show that the proportion of households that go hungry has declined from 17.3 percent in 1983 to 2.5 percent in 2004-05. However in spite of the problems of overestimation with this data as is based on self-perception by the head of the household, there has been a perceptible decline in hunger to different degrees in various states. However poverty levels are still high in the country due to the lack of economic access to food at the household level.

Apart from the overall levels of hunger reported in the country, access to food is also to varying degrees reflected by poverty ratios, the levels of employment and access to the PDS. Each of these indicators will be briefly analyzed to get an overall perception of the access to food (physical and economic).

Household Food Security: Poverty Levels

The incidence of poverty does indicate the extent to which food is accessible. The expenditure on food along with some provision for non-food expenditure is normally used to estimate the poverty line.

According to official estimates, there has been a significant reduction in the population below the poverty line. While there were 55 percent of households below the poverty line in 1970, this came down to 28 percent in 2004-05. However over 300 million people still languish below the official poverty line. Though there is a little agreement on the official methodology of estimating the poverty line, increase in inequality does seem to have been arrested to some extent. It is further seen that the extent of poverty reduction was much lower in the first half of the reforms period (1993-2000) as compared to the second half (1999-2005). This may have been due to lower food prices, and higher employment in the non-farm sector during the later half of the reforms decade though the growth in the agricultural sector was significantly lower during this later half. It is now clear on the basis of estimated poverty ratios that there is no significant decline in poverty during the period after economic reforms were initiated as compared to the pre-reform period wherein growth was reported to be much lower. It is also unambiguously clear that inequality increased significantly in the period after reforms as compared to the pre-reform period. It is also observed that there is a concentration in poverty in some regions as well as among some vulnerable groups such as the Schedule Caste and Schedule Tribes.

Though there has been an overall decline in poverty in the post Independence era, some specific states still have a high poverty ratio. The poverty ratio in Bihar, Odisha, Chhattisgarh and Jharkhand was in excess of 40 percent in 2004-05 while it was between 30 and 40 percent in states such as Madhya Pradesh, Uttarakhand and Uttar Pradesh.

State level estimates clearly show an increasing concentration of the poor in a few states (Radhakrishna and Ray, 2005). It is also seen that in a group of four states namely Bihar, Madhya Pradesh, Odisha and Uttar Pradesh, the share of the rural poor in the country already stood at 49.8

percent in 1983. This share increased to 55 percent in 1993-94 and further to a high level of 61 percent in the year 2004-05. Moreover, poverty in the case of the total population is seen to be concentrated in five states namely Bihar, Madhya Pradesh, Odisha, Maharashtra, and Uttar Pradesh and their share of the total poor in 2004-05 stood at 65 percent.

Figures in Table 7 complied by the Planning Commission shown that poverty is getting concentrated among SCs and STs in some of the poorer states. It is seen that rural poverty among these groups was as high as 76 percent in Odisha while it was as high as 64 percent in Bihar during the year 2004-05. The case of urban poverty is quite similar for SCs and STs during the year 2004-05.

Table 7: Poverty Ratios by Selected Groups in Selected States.

Year	Rural			Urban		
	SC	ST	OBC	SC	ST	OBC
Bihar	64.0	53.3	37.8	67.2	57.2	41.4
Chhattisgarh	32.7	54.7	33.9	52.0	41.0	52.7
Jharkhand	57.9	54.2	40.2	47.2	45.1	19.1
M.P.	42.8	58.6	29.6	67.3	44.7	55.5
Maharashtra	44.8	56.6	23.9	43.2	40.4	35.6
Odisha	50.2	75.6	36.9	72.6	61.8	50.2
Uttarakhand	54.2	43.2	44.8	65.7	64.4	46.5
All India	36.8	47.3	26.7	39.9	33.3	31.4

Source: Planning Commission, GoI, 2009

If one goes by the poverty estimates arrived at by the Expert Group on Methodology for Estimation of Poverty (GoI, 2009) and often referred to as the Tendulkar Committee Report, the overall poverty ratio in India was 37.2 percent. The rural and urban poverty ratios at the all India level were 41.8 percent and 25.7 percent respectively. Based on these estimates the absolute number of the poor in India was more than 400 million in 2004-05 a level that is still far from acceptable.

The effective reduction in poverty hinges on much higher growth in agriculture as well as in the non-farm rural sector. This growth needs to be accompanied by a reduction in rural-urban disparities across regions as well as an effective reduction in social disparities that are disturbing. It is important to mention here that the recent increases in food prices should be a major cause for concern in the context of the present poverty levels and is likely to have caused serious inroads in the access to food for the poverty groups.

The Growth in Employment

The sustained creation of employment goes a long way in effectively increasing access and ensuring the right to food. The increase in employment opportunities especially for the poor enables them to obtain the purchasing power to increase their food consumption. The overall growth in employment in the country is thus closely related to the ability to improve access to food particularly for the poor in both rural and urban India.

It is seen in Table 8 that the employment growth rate has been relatively higher in the urban economy as compared to the rural sector during the period from 1983 to 2004-05. The rate of growth in employment is reported to have declined in the post-reform period of 1993-94 to 2004-05. The decline was seen to be greater in the rural sector than in urban areas. It is also seen that male employment did grow at a faster rate as compared to female employment, however the gap between the two was much smaller in the post-reform period of 1993-94 and 2004-05. It is also interesting to see that female employment grew at a higher rate during this period indicating that more women entered the labour force in general and particularly in the rural areas indicating a feminization of farming activity with women having to participate in order to supplement the effort of men. The significant overall decline in the growth rate of employment in the post-reform period as compared to the pre-reform period indicates a disturbing trend and thus indicates a decline in the ability to access food due to lower purchasing power.

Table 8: Growth Rates of Employment, 1983 to 2005

Growth of Employment			
	Male	Female	Total
1983-94	2.25	1.65	2.08
1994-2005	1.87	1.78	1.84
	Rural		
1983-94	1.96	1.40	1.77
1994-2005	1.41	1.55	1.46
	Urban		
1983-94	3.15	3.37	3.26
1994-2005	3.10	3.08	3.09

Source: Estimates of S. Mahendra Dev and A. Sharma, 2010, using NSS data.

Since agricultural wages is an indicator of purchasing power a healthy growth in real agricultural wages assists in the reduction of poverty in rural areas and leads to greater access to food and other essential needs (Deaton and Dreze, 2002). Though the growth in both the regular and casual wage has been constant in rural areas it is reported that real wages has declined substantially during the later half of the reforms period (S. Mahendra Dev and A. Sharma, 2010).

Turning to the plight of landless labourers it is seen that the growth rate of employment has slowed down considerably and unemployment among agricultural labour households has increased from 9.5 percent in 1993-94 to as much as 15.3 percent in 2004-05.

According to the NSS data, the proportion of landless households as a proportion of all households has increased from 25.1 percent in 1973-74 to 38.7 percent in 1993-94 and further to as high as 43.1 percent in 2004-05 with such increases in the supply of labour there has been a notable decline in the rate of growth in real wages of adult casual labourers which has seen a declining trend (Jha, Praveen. 2007).

Access to the Public Distribution System

The long established PDS has played a vital role in partially meeting the essential food and fuel needs of households in India. The operation of the PDS is supplementary in nature and does not meet the entire food requirements of any household however it does effectively protect the household by providing a basic entitlement at affordable prices and at convenient locations through its wide network of Fair Price Shops.

The proportion of food grains accessed through the PDS in the total household consumption provides an indicator of the effectiveness of the PDS in ensuring food security in India. As seen in Table 9 that at the national level the consumption requirement met through the PDS by households has increased significantly during the period 1993-94 to 2009-10. However there are wide interstate variations reflecting the fact that the PDS has performed much better in meeting household requirements in some states as compared to others. The share of the PDS in the total consumption of both rice and wheat is seen to be much higher in Andhra Pradesh, Chhattisgarh, Himachal Pradesh, Jammu and Kashmir, Karnataka, Kerala, Odisha and Tamil Nadu. In these states the PDS appears to be functioning well and providing access to households. (Anjani, Kumar. et al. 2012)

It is also seen in Table 9 that the PDS in states such as Assam, Bihar and Uttar Pradesh have not performed well and provided limited access to households. The PDS in these states require to be made more effective as these states account for a large population of poor households who still lack access to affordable food grain. However in general the penetration of the PDS has increased in most states over the time and the share of household requirements of food grain accessed has improved though to varying degrees. The PDS has thus proved to be one of the most effective policy instruments in providing greater access and food security. The increased supply of food grains to the rural areas has also contributed to crop diversification especially in the southern, western and the northeastern regions. Though the system is poorly targeted and suffers from widespread leakages and the diversion of grain to the open market it has still gone a long way in protecting and covering a large number of poor consumers. With the proposed NFSA, the improved functioning of the PDS would become most essential and concerted efforts would have to be made in effectively plugging leakages and ensuring a streamlined functioning of the PDS.

Table 9: The Share of the PDS in Rice and Wheat Consumption in Different States, 1993-94 to 2009-10

State	Rice		Wheat		Rice and Wheat	
	1993-1994	2009-2010	1993-1994	2009-2010	1993-1994	2009-2010
Andhra Pradesh	20.6	29.7	9.1	4.0	20.4	28.5
Assam	3.2	10.4	2.7	1.3	3.1	10.0
Bihar	0.2	4.7	0.3	4.8	0.3	4.7
Chhattisgarh	2.2	38.8	2.4	28.7	2.3	37.7
Gujarat	20.1	13.7	0.4	10.5	6.6	11.4
Haryana	4.3	0.5	0.0	12.4	0.4	11.4
Himachal Pradesh	32.5	43.3	0.3	44.3	12.3	43.9
Jammu & Kashmir	5.5	53.4	0.3	32.5	2.2	46.9
Jharkhand	0.3	12.7	1.9	15.4	0.7	13.5
Karnataka	14.5	34.5	1.4	26.1	12.5	32.9
Kerala	44.4	26.2	13.7	27.1	41.8	26.3
Madhya Pradesh	3.6	17.2	0.2	19.7	2.0	19.2
Maharashtra	13.4	22.4	0.3	21.4	7.2	21.8
Odisha	0.8	22.9	5.1	12.6	0.9	22.3
Punjab	2.3	0.1	0.1	12.7	0.3	11.5
Rajasthan	7.4	0.3	0.1	9.3	0.3	9.0
Tamil Nadu	17.9	47.6	2.8	51.8	17.1	47.9
Uttar Pradesh	3.2	16.1	0.0	6.8	0.9	10.0
Uttarakhand	45.9	19.6	0.2	13.2	20.6	16.0
West Bengal	1.7	5.3	2.0	28.3	1.7	8.3
All India	9.9	21.7	0.4	12.7	6.0	17.8

Source: Estimates of Anjani Kumar et al., 2012, using NSS data.

The Trends and Performance in Nutrition Indicators

The adequacy of food and nutrition and the proper assessment of inadequate food intake among individuals and population groups are usually based on the Nutritional Intake Assessment as well as the assessment of Nutritional Status.

Nutritional Intake of Calories, Protein and Fat

The trends in the per capita calorie, protein and fat intake of the population are often used in assessing the adequacy of food and nutrition. These figures are presented in Table 10, and pertain to the period starting from 1983-84 to 2009-10. These trends have been computed separately for the rural as well as the urban population.

Table 10: Mean Per Capita Consumption of Calories, Protein and Fats for Rural and Urban Households in India

(per capita/day)

Year	Calories (kcal)		Protein (gms)		Fats (gms)	
	Rural	Urban	Rural	Urban	Rural	Urban
1983-84	2240	2070	63.5	58.1	27.1	37.1
1987-88	2233	2095	63.2	58.6	28.3	39.3
1993-94	2153	2073	60.3	57.7	31.1	41.9
1999-00	2148	2155	59.1	58.4	36.0	49.6
2004-05	2047	2021	55.8	55.4	35.4	47.4
2009-10	2147	2123	59.3	58.8	43.1	53.0

Source: *NSSO reports* (various rounds)

As seen in Table 10 the pattern of calorie and protein intake for rural and urban households show a dissimilar trend during the period 1983-84 to 2009-10 while per capita calorie intake declined from a level of 2240 kcal per day in 1983-84 to 2147 kcal per day in 2009-10, for the rural population. The per capita protein intake for the rural population declined from 63.5 gm to 59 gm per day during the same period. The per capita calorie intake for the urban population however increased marginally from 2070 kcal per day to 2123 kcal per day and per capita protein intake from 58.1 gm per day to 58.8 gm per day in the period between 1983-84 and 2009-10. On the other hand the per capita intake of fat increased steadily over time for both rural and urban population.

The decline in calorie intake among the rural population has been attributed by some scholars to the lowering of energy requirement that result from a sedentary lifestyle, increasing mechanization of agricultural activities and the use of mechanized transport. However these arguments fail on the basis of the significant rise in calorie intake reported between 2004-05 and 2009-10 for the rural population.

These arguments can also be refuted on the basis of figures of the per capita calorie and protein intake for the poor and rich households for the period 1983-84 to 2009-10 as given in Table 11. It is seen here that in the case of poor households the calorie intake was much lower than the rich and its increase over the period was negligible though it did fluctuate significantly in between.

Table 11: Trends in the Per Capita Intake of Calorie, Protein and Fat by the Poor and Rich Households in India

(per capita per day)

Year(TE)	Calorie (kcal)		Protein (gms)		Fat (gms)	
	Poor	Rich	Poor	Rich	Poor	Rich
1983	1698	2747	48	77	17	48
1987-88	1754	2791	50	80	19	52
1993-94	1544	2327	42	65	20	52
1999-00	1670	2756	45	73	22	71
2004-05	1757	2636	44	66	23	53
2009-10	1754	2819	48	85	29	71

Source: Estimates of Anjani Kumar et al., 2012,

What seems clearly evident is the glaring difference between the calorie and protein intake between the poor and rich households. This is more disturbing as the intake for the poor is still far below the prescribed norms. There has thus been stagnation if not a decline in the per capita calorie and protein intake among the poor rural households reflecting a very low nutritional intake.

Nutritional Status

We now turn our attention to nutritional status especially among the most vulnerable groups namely women and children. The National Nutritional Monitoring Bureau provides the nutritional status of rural households in nine sampled states. The report categories children in the age group of 1 to 5 years into different nutritional grades based on weight for age. The data thus classified indicates that the proportion of underweight children declined significantly from a level of 77 percent in 1975-79 to 55 percent in 2004-05.

The data provided by the National Family Health Survey (NFHS) indicates that the proportion of underweight children declined marginally from 47 percent in 1998-99 to 45.9 percent in 2005-06 although stunting among children declined more impressively. What is perhaps more disturbing however is that the percentage of children reported to be wasted in 1998-99 was 15.5 percent but this figure increased to 19.1 percent in 2005-06 as seen in Table 12 below.

Table 12: Trends in Child Malnutrition (0-3 years)

Nutritional Parameter	1992-93 NFHS-1	1998-99 NFHS-2	2005-06 NFHS-3
Stunted	52.0	45.5	38.4
Wasted	17.5	15.5	19.1
Underweight	53.4	47.0	45.9

Source: Factsheets NFHS-1, 2, & 3

It may also be mentioned that while the rate of decline in child malnutrition is expected to be around half the rate of growth of per capita GDP in most developing countries the situation is not so in India where the rate of decline in malnutrition is much lower than per capita income growth. It is also seen on the basis of data from the Family Health Surveys that the level of malnutrition among children is much higher in rural areas as compared to urban areas.

Turning to the incidence of malnutrition among vulnerable groups of women it is seen in Table 13 below that at all India level the incidence of malnutrition among women is the highest for Scheduled Castes and Scheduled Tribes followed by women belonging to other Backward Communities and Muslims. At the level of individual states malnutrition among women is the highest in states such as Bihar, Chhattisgarh, Jharkhand, Madhya Pradesh and below, while it is the lowest in States such as Punjab and Kerala as seen in Table 13 below.

Indicators on anemia for women and children provided by the NFHS-III show that more than 50 percent of women and nearly 80 percent of children are victims of anemia, this reflects a very high level of micronutrient deficiencies that have very adverse effects on maternal and child health.

4. POLICIES AND PROGRAMMES FOR IMPROVING ACCESS AND NUTRITION

Access to food is determined by increases in purchasing power brought about by rising employment and supported by social protection programmes. However factors affecting malnutrition are far more varied and complex as compared to those that affected access to food though the both closely interrelated. Here we discuss the factors that influence access and nutrition and the policies pursued to improve these two important aspects of food security.

Table 13: Incidence of Malnutrition among Women 2005-06

State	Total Population	SC/ST Population	OBC Population	Muslim Population	Others
India	35.6	42.7	36.0	35.1	27.5
Andhra Pradesh	33.5	38.4	37.0	27.6	22.2
Assam	36.5	34.5	30.4	46.0	31.4
Bihar	45.1	58.4	43.3	49.6	31.4
Chhattisgarh	43.4	46.6	44.8	28.9	26.2
Gujarat	36.3	48.0	40.5	37.0	22.9
Haryana	31.3	36.4	33.1	49.0	26.6
Jharkhand	43.0	44.6	45.3	47.3	26.5
Karnataka	35.5	41.8	34.9	26.9	31.7
Kerala	18.0	24.1	18.6	15.6	18.0
Madhya Pradesh	41.7	48.7	42.2	37.4	27.7
Maharashtra	36.2	43.6	36.1	23.8	34.5
Odisha	41.4	50.6	39.6	63.5	30.7
Punjab	18.9	26.7	18.0	22.5	14.4
Rajasthan	36.7	44.1	33.3	36.1	32.3
Tamil Nadu	28.4	36.1	26.8	20.7	8.3
Uttar Pradesh	36.4	43.6	35.4	36.4	28.3
West Bengal	39.1	45.2	39.2	37.4	31.5

Source: S. Mahendra Dev, and A. Sharma 2010, and based on NFHS-3 data.

Growth in Incomes, Access to Food and Nutrition

Growth in incomes not only enhances greater access to food but can improve nutrition as well. It has been seen, as mentioned earlier that the decline in malnutrition comes about with the rise in per capita incomes. It is further observed that the percentage decline in malnutrition is about half the rate of per capita growth in most countries. However, this will only happen if growth is equitable. In recent times we have witnessed the GDP growing in India by 6 to 7 percent, however the percentage decline in child malnutrition has declined by only 0.5 percent per annum. Iniquitous or non-inclusive growth that predominantly benefits the rich and not the poor largely explains the much slower decline in malnutrition. Economic growth alone cannot reduce malnutrition as other enabling factors play an equally important role. Income growth is thus necessary but not a sufficient condition in the effective reduction in malnutrition.

Income poverty is yet another reason for lack of access to food and malnutrition. However many studies have indicated that malnutrition continues to exist even after poverty has been eradicated. While income poverty in India is about 27 percent child malnutrition continues to persist at a high level of 46 percent.

There is, however, no denying the fact that income growth can reduce malnutrition. It is seen on the basis of NFHS-II data, that in 2005-06 while proportion of undernourished children stood at 56.6 percent for the poorest households it still persisted to be as high as 19.7 percent for the wealthiest households.

Determinants of Malnutrition

The three major factors that influence the level of nutrition in most developing countries are (*i*) household food security (caused by low availability and access) (*ii*) inadequate maternal care and child care practices (*iii*) lack of healthcare services, clean drinking water and sanitation; and (iv) high gender inequality. There are both direct as well as indirect or institutional determinants of under nutrition. While food and micronutrient intake, diet diversification, health services, water and sanitation are direct factors, women empowerment and gender equality, agricultural growth and expansion of the rural non-farm sector are indirect or institutional factors.

Adequacy of Food Intake and Diversification of Diets

The consumption of adequate food containing the required calorie, proteins and micronutrients is necessary for combating malnutrition. There is a need to shift one"s focus on providing a range of food, which is rich in essential micronutrients, energy and the required protein. A diversified diet that takes care of the balanced nutritional needs especially of the vulnerable population, which faces the constant risk of malnutrition, needs to be effectively implemented in the case of various feeding programmes such as the ICDS and the MDMS.

Public Health

The state of public health services is far from satisfactory. These suffer from significant regional, social disparities, and gender disparities reflecting low levels of health indicators, which have hardly improved over the years. The quality of delivery systems is very poor. There has also been significant privatization of health services that are unaffordable and expensive, impacting very adversely on the poor who are as a result forced to compromise other essential expenditures such as on food and education. The low standards of health, hygiene, safe drinking water and sanitation play a very adverse role by inhibiting the absorption of essential nutrients by children who are sick and ailing. There is thus a crying need for larger investments in public healthcare and its radical improvement.

Empowerment of Women

It is now widely accepted that an improvement in the status of women, and their well-being would in turn significantly improve the well-being of children. The mechanisms through which women"s empowerment is effectively transferred to the well being of the child are maternal education, economic empowerment, and the power to make decisions within the household and empowerment of women in the community. The improvement in the status of women in the community also helps them in articulating and even demanding better child related services (Jones et al, 2007).

The level of child nutrition is determined by the capacity of mothers to take care of the child"s needs. Caring capacity and practices are significantly influenced by the status of women in the household and in society at large.

The adequate nutrition of women during pregnancy is critical for its impact on birth weight. Malnourished mothers are more likely to give birth to low birth weight babies who are most likely to be stunted and undernourished. Poor pre-natal nutritional status of the mother leads to inadequate breast-feeding. Poorly educated mothers are most likely to ignore supplementary feeding and children are often denied of sufficient quality food during the first two years that is most essential to ensure normal mental and physical abilities as the child grows.

Multi-Sectoral Interventions

There is a pressing need to ensure coordinated interventions on several fronts such as processes for improving clean drinking water, sanitation and public hygiene, elementary education, immunization, antenatal care and nutritional supplementation. A package of such interventions will bring about lower child mortality and child nutrition. The need to achieve a high level of synergy between sectors is thus most essential.

Agricultural Growth and Development

Among the other indirect or institutional factors that impact the level of nutrition is the diversified growth and development of the agricultural sector. This sector not only ensures better food availability but can also increase access to food and nutrition. It is seen that agricultural growth is slow in States where malnutrition is high in the central and eastern states. The increased involvement of women in raising home gardens and the incorporation of nutritional elements in crop production and diversification can tackle the problems of malnutrition to a significant extent.

The Non-Farm Sector

With a very large proportion of the workers engaged in and dependent on agriculture, the scope of further expansion of livelihoods based on agriculture alone is limited. There is thus a need to expend the rural non-farm sector to provide greater earning opportunities for those confined to agriculture.

Food processing and other services such as storage, transport and marketing need to be encouraged through higher outlays and investments in rural non-farm infrastructure.

Social Protection Programmes

Well-designed and effectively implemented social protection programmes are essential for ensuring access to food and comprehensively addressing the problem of malnutrition. These programmes are non-contributory and sharply targeted transfer programmes that focus on the poor and vulnerable sections of the population. A purely market oriented growth strategy is incapable of effectively reducing risks and inequality. The state has to step in and maintain social cohesion and avoid irreversible losses in human capital. The state plays a vital role especially in times of insecurity by ensuring the required minimum level of provisioning for those that are excluded from the growth process. Among the many social protection programmes in India there are two broad categories specifically targeted for the poor and closely related to food security and nutrition. These are (*i*) The Public Distribution System and Supplementary Nutrition Programmes and (*ii*) The Rural Wage Employment Programme. In what follows we shall examine these programmes and also suggest specific measures to improve the effectiveness and impact of these schemes.

The Targeted Public Distribution System

The Public Distribution System is designed to improve food security at the household level in India. The PDS provides commodities like rice, wheat, sugar, edible oils and kerosene to identified and registered beneficiaries through a network of dedicated retail outlets, known as fair price shops at fixed prices that are normally lower than open market prices. The PDS with its national network of over 4.5 lakh fair price shops and distributing commodities worth more than Rs 300 billion annually to about 160 million households is perhaps the largest distribution network in the world. It has evolved over many decades as a vital instrument of food policy in India for coping with scarcities, controlling prices of essential commodities in the open market and ensuring physical availability of essential supplies at affordable prices for the poor. The scheme however is supplemental in nature and is not intended to provide the entire requirements of households.

The presently operating Targeted Public Distribution System (TPDS) caters to all households in India and can thus be said to have universal coverage. However these households/beneficiaries are treated differently on the basis of their income. The entire household population is broadly classified into two income groups, those above the officially accepted poverty line are categorized as above poverty line or APL households; and those households below the poverty line or BPL households. Moreover there exists a sub-category of the BPL households who constitute the "poorest of the poor" and who are categorized as the Antyodaya Anna Yojana (AAY) households consisting of the old and destitute population usually uncared for and abandoned by the younger members of the family. Left to fend for themselves they are most vulnerable requiring special treatment and assistance. The AAY category is thus provided their entitlements at specially subsidized prices, which are considerably lower than the subsidized prices fixed for the BPL households.

While the APL group is provided a fixed monthly entitlement at prices that cover „economic costs" thereby not involving any subsidy, the BPL households are provided a monthly entitlement of 35 kg of cereals and a fixed monthly entitlement of other essential commodities such as sugar and K-oil at subsidized prices significantly lower than economic cost. The AAY beneficiaries are also provided a fixed entitlement of 35 kg of food grain at specially subsidized rates of Rs 2 per kg of wheat and Rs 3 per kg of rice. It is important to mention that all the different household categories of beneficiaries covered by the TPDS are effectively protected from open market prices, which normally rule at higher levels as compared to economic cost.

Under the distribution system food grains and other essential commodities are allocated to the state governments on the basis of officially accepted poverty ratios. According to these accepted poverty ratios, the Central Government estimates that there are as many as 65 million poor households in the country spread over different states and Union Territories. The states in turn distribute the Centrally allocated food grains according to its BPL list. There is a problem here as the BPL list of most states adds up to a 100 million poor households far in excess of the estimates provided by the Central Government.

The glaring discrepancy is entirely on account of the different methodology followed by the Central and state governments for estimating the number of BPL households in a state. This intractable problem can only be solved if a common methodology agreed upon by both the Central Government and the states is used for the identification of beneficiaries, as the „errors of inclusion" can be as important as the „errors of exclusion" in order to ensure effective targeting.

Major Concerns Regarding the PDS and Suggestions for Improving it's Functioning

One of the major problems of the PDS is its penetration and effectiveness to reach the target groups in most parts of the country. Access is thus limited and it is able to meet only a limited proportion of the monthly food grain consumption. Although its effectiveness in the Southern and North Eastern States has improved over the years, it has hardly made any impact in some of the poorer States such as Bihar, Assam and Uttar Pradesh and displays marked regional disparities.

The reports of the High Level Committee on Long-term Grain Policy (GoI: 2002) and the Performance Evaluation of the Targeted Public Distribution System (PEO, Planning Commission, 2005) have highlighted some major problems in the present TPDS. These are high exclusion errors due to the improper identification of beneficiaries, the non-viability of fair price shops, its inability to effectively carry out the price stabilization function and high levels of leakages and diversion of grain to the open market. There are yet other discrepancies in the distribution system such as irregular and infrequent supply of food grains by fair price shops, the inefficiency of the Food Corporation of India, the lack of a proper system of inspection of entitlements, low margins and lack of profitability for fair price shops.

Suggestions for Improvement

There are several measures that are required to be taken for improving the effectiveness of the procurement and distribution system. The most critical among these are:

1. The decentralization of procurement and distribution has become necessary to improve and strengthen the PDS.

2. A greater and more active involvement of the panchayats in the PDS can significantly improve access at the village level.

3. A comprehensive review of the functioning of the FCI and the modernization of its operations is overdue and the greater involvement of cooperatives, self help groups, and other community organizations in procurement as well as distribution should be a top priority.

4. Improving the turnover and margins of fair price shops, provision of credit to enable regular lifting and sale of supplies, and the regular monitoring of retail sales is necessary for effectively tackling and plugging diversion as well as other malpractices such as adulteration.

5. Concerted efforts are needed for computerization of records, and the issue of smart cards to beneficiaries is essential for greater accountability and transparency.

6. Evolving a comprehensive criterion for the selection of agencies and individuals for retail FPS operation, and the strictest enforcement of these criteria would significantly improve effectiveness of the retail network.

7. Improving storage space, and the introduction of properly and regularly calibrated weighing equipment in fair price shops has become essential both for maintaining regular and uninterrupted supplies and efficient sale.

8. There is also an urgent need to set up a proper and effective grievances redressal system for both the fair price shops as well as beneficiaries.

9. There is also an urgent need to enforce appropriate penalties and punishment for defaulters.

10. The bar coding of bags containing the food grain and sugar released by the FCI will go a long way in tracking movement of supplies right down to the retail or FPS level, and also effectively check the diversion of supplies. The inspectorate has to be appropriately equipped with the means of modern mobile surveillance for enhanced monitoring and vigilance.

11. The number of retail outlets should be seriously reviewed by each state government and the emphasis should be on an appropriate number of well equipped and financially viable fair price shops rather than a proliferation of non-functional outlets supposedly licensed for providing location convenience to beneficiaries.

Nutrition Programmes

The Integrated Child Development Services (ICDS) and the Mid-day Meal Scheme (MDMS) are two major initiatives for improving the level of nutrition. These programmes are well established, popular, and comprehensively designed. These schemes have universal coverage and cater to the entire population in all regions and states.

The Integrated Child Development Services (ICDS)

The main objective of the ICDS is the holistic development of children up to the age of six years with a very special focus on children up to the age of two years. It also caters to expectant and locating mothers. These objectives are attempted to be achieved through the provision of a package of services such as basic health check-ups, immunization, referral services, supplementary feeding, non-formal pre-school education, and the required advice on essential health practices and nutrition. These services are made available through a wide network of childcare centres popularly known as „Anganwadis". In spite of its expansion and popularity over the last three decades its impact has been limited. It is seen that the problem of child and maternal malnutrition still persists. Child malnutrition has not declined significantly and it is reported that anemia among children and women has increased with as many as one-third of all adult women being undernourished. The services have also had a limited coverage and outreach. The solution thus lies in increasing its coverage to ensure effective universalization, changing and improving its design, and planning its effective implementation in order to achieve its objectives (GoI, 2008).

Measures to Improve the ICDS

A very comprehensive set of suggestions for the improvement of ICDS has been made by N.C. Saxena, an experienced civil servant and renowned scholar (Saxena N.C., 2011). These suggestions, which are very comprehensive as well as administratively feasible, are as follows:

Malnutrition starts to set in quite fast among children aged six to twelve months and adequate precautions need to be taken at an early stage. It is thus suggested that the focus should now shift to children aged less than two years. There should be increased spending on infant and young child nutrition during the first 24 months when malnutrition is most frequent and adversely affects the very foundations of life and development. Increased targets for breast-feeding should be set for each centre and closely monitored by independent sources.

Proper rehabilitation facilities similar to the Nutrition Rehabilitation Centres should be made available at the PHCs at the district level and ICDS workers should be made responsible for identifying children and mothers suffering severe malnutrition and referring them to these centres.

Each centre must have the necessary minimum infrastructure and equipment for providing effective services. A proper guideline for infrastructure should be evolved and a checklist of facilities which include proper weighing and measuring scales, storage facilities, drinking water, child friendly toilets, medicine kits and a separate kitchen shed should be prepared.

Two freshly cooked meals (breakfast and lunch) should be provided. This food should be prepared under hygienic conditions and proper supervision. Prepared at the anganwadi, the meals should be based on locally available nutritious ingredients. The supply of packaged foods must be avoided as it is not popular with children and their procurement is likely to lead to various kinds of corruption and diversion.

For children who are below the age of three years take home rations (THR) should be provided. These rations should be carefully composed, locally procured and prepared. Weaning foods are also essential and the budget for this should be significantly increased.

Supplementary feeding should be accompanied by proper nutritional counseling, adequate nutrition and health education and simple home based interventions such as always boiling drinking water. These are essential for ensuring infection free growth and development.

The programme needs local involvement and control to maintain and sustain services of good quality. It is therefore essential to involve the active participation and control of panchayats and other community groups. States must ensure that the anganwadi workers are selected out of eligible persons by the gramsabha; it would also be desirable to appoint local persons who would be accountable and regular in her duties.

A comprehensive criteria needs to be evolved for the grading and accreditation of anganwadi centres. This should be coordinated by the panchayat and involve the participation of mothers committees and community groups. Accreditation can be used to provide rewards and incentives for performance. This will also attract more young mothers and their children to participate in the programme and enhance its outreach and coverage while inducing other centres to improve their status and performance.

A special component should be included and expanded catering to the special need of adolescent girls. They should be universally screened and periodically weighed. There progress should be closely monitored and evaluated according to three age groups namely girls in the 10-15 age group, those between 16-19 years, and those who are pregnant. They should also be provided with the appropriate food that contains essential micronutrients and iron. Similar services should be provided to all women in their childbearing age.

Children of migrant workers should not be excluded from ICDS and they should be admitted and be allowed to use all the services provided in the ICDS. Data should also be disaggregated at the ICDS level for enrollment and actual coverage, to reflect the number and proportion of disabled children and of children from vulnerable local SC and ST communities. Exclusion of children from vulnerable communities is unacceptable and should be panelized.

State governments should be firmly directed to cover all urban slums within a period of two years. Prefabricated structures should be developed to enable the programme to function in unauthorized slum settlements or construction and brick kiln sites. In rural areas ICDS centres on a priority basis should be set up within a year in all Primitive Tribal Group Settlements and marginalized SC settlements without any minimum ceiling on the number of children they contain. The same is suggested for all other hamlets with more than 50 percent SCs, STs or minority population within a maximum of two years. In all these centres ICDS staff should be local to the relevant communities and two hot meals should be served instead of one to children aged three to six years with double weaning food provided to children under three. These specially located ICDS centres should extend their nutrition and health services to all categories of single women and not restrict these services to only expectant and lactating mothers as presently practiced in the programme.

The Mid Day Meal Scheme (MDMS)

This scheme provides a free cooked meal to primary school children of government, government aided and schools run by local bodies. This scheme is Centrally assisted with the State Governments making some contributions towards the cost of cooking the meal provided.

The MDMS launched in 1995 with the Central Government providing free foodgrains while the costs of cooking the meal was entirely borne by the state governments. However, due to inadequate funding, some state governments resorted to distributing foodgrains instead of providing cooked mid day meals. Under the orders of Supreme Court, the scheme was revised as well as universalized in 2004 to provide a cooked mid day meal containing atleast 300 calories and 8 to 12 grams of protein to all children in the government and government aided primary schools. The scheme was extended to upper primary schools from October 2007.

Though the scheme is considered to be popular and successful, it is faced with several problems. In 2005-06, of the grain allocated by the Central Governments based on estimates of enrollments and attendance, the state governments lifted only 76,8 percent. This implies that either all the institutions or children entitled to the MDM were not fully covered. It could also imply that providing insufficient quantity of food compromised the stipulated quality of the meal or it could also mean that meals were not provided on all working days. The problem faced by the scheme thus mainly relate to quality, quantity and irregularity of the mid day meal that is provided to children.

The other important problems relating to the scheme were reflected in the performance audit report on the Mid Day Meal Scheme by the CAG of India (CAG: 2008). This report found that many states resort to over reporting the enrolment while estimating their demand for funds. The report mentions that there is no system of cross checking the enrolment data furnished by the state governments. It was also indicated that in most states children were not provided micronutrient supplements or de-worming medicines.

The provision for the regular monitoring and evaluation as well as inspections in the scheme designed were not effectively followed nor any lessons learned and measures initiated to correct the observed flaws. It was also reported that the undesirable involvement of teachers in supervising the cooking and serving of the meal resulted in detraction from their teaching responsibilities through less of teaching hours. The other problems that the scheme is faced with are the lack of adequate infrastructure for the clean and hygienic functioning of the programme, improper and unsafe storage of food and other cooking ingredients, as well as low and adulterated quality of materials used. This serious neglect of quality and hygiene has recently even led to the sickness and death of school children.

Suggestions for Improving the MDMS

Keeping in mind the various flaws and shortcomings of this important nutritional intervention, the following suggestions are being made for its improvement.

The local community, the PRIs and NGOs, must manage the MDMS and should not be contractor-driven.

Sensitize senior teachers and supervisory staff on nutrition, hygiene, and cleanliness and safety norms so that the defects are detected and corrected promptly.

Nutrition experts should be required to plan low cost nutritionally balanced menu and for periodic testing of samples of prepared food.

Promote the use of locally grown and procured nutritionally rich food items such as leafy vegetables and pulses. This may be supplemented by promoting kitchen gardens in the school premises with the active assistance and support of the concerned state government, department or line agency.

The provision of cooking costs should be increased to Rs 3 per child and this revised norm must be inflation-linked so that it is constantly reviewed.

Proper infrastructure for the MDMS should be mandatory, including cooking sheds, storage space, clean drinking water and proper cooking utensils.

The MDMS should be integrated with the school health services and must include immunization, de-worming, growth monitoring, health check-ups and micronutrient supplementation.

Active community participation in vigilance and monitoring of the MDMS must be encouraged and strengthened in order to prevent corruption and ensure quality. The involvement of the panchayat and local parents must be ensured in this regard.

Status regarding supplies, available funds, stipulated norms and the weekly menu must be mandatorily and prominently displayed in order to be inspected by anyone who wishes to. This will ensure a high level of transparency regarding the programme.

In the event of any act of social discrimination in the MDMS, which may be detected or reported to the authorities, serious and prompt action must be taken after due and proper investigation by a competent authority.

The regular social audit of the MDMS and its concurrent monitoring by independent agencies must be carried out.

The National Rural Employment Guarantee Programme

Rural works programmes are now widely recognized as important instruments in the strategy for poverty alleviation and hunger through employment generation. They enhance the purchasing capacity and this is expected to increase the access to food.

The Mahatma Gandhi National Rural Employment Guarantee Act, 2005 (MGNREGA) was notified in September 2005. The Act"s mandate is to provide at least 100 days of guaranteed wage employment in a financial year to every rural household whose adult members volunteer to do unskilled manual work.

The major goals of the Act are:

To provide social protection to the most vulnerable people living in rural India by providing employment opportunities.

Livelihood security for the poor through the creation of durable assets, improved water security, soil conservation and higher land productivity.

Drought proofing and flood management in rural India.

Empowerment of the socially disadvantaged especially women, SCs and STs through the processes of a rights-based legislation.

Strengthening decentralized participatory planning through the convergence of various anti-poverty and livelihood initiatives.

Deepening democracy at the grassroots by strengthening Panchayati Raj Institutions.

Bringing about greater transparency and accountability in governance.

The MGNREGA is thus a powerful instrument for ensuring inclusive growth in rural India through its impact on social protection, democratic empowerment and livelihood security.

The Act was initially notified in a limited number of districts but at present extended to all districts in the country with the exception of those that have an entirely urban population.

The MGNREGA is the largest employment programme in the world unlike any other wage employment programme in its scale and architecture. Its bottom-up, demand-driven, self-targeted and rights-based design is unprecedented. The Act ensures a legal guarantee for unskilled wage employment. Work is provided by the demand for work by wage seekers and not on any other consideration. The Act also provides legal provisions and allowances for failure to provide work on demand and also for delay in payment of wages.

Moreover the Act overcomes problems related to identification and targeting as it is a self-targeting scheme and covers all who demand and volunteer to undertake unskilled manual labour. The Act also incentivises the states to provide work as 100 percent of the unskilled labour cost and 75 percent of the skilled labour costs and material costs are provided by the Centre. There is also a disincentive for failing to provide work, as the state has to then bear the cost of the unemployment allowance that is mandatorily provided for. With gram panchayats required to implement at least 50 percent of all works in terms of cost, there is a very high degree of financial devolution. The plan and decisions regarding the nature and choice of works, the order in which each work is to be carried out, and decisions on site selection is decentralized and decided by the gram sabha. Finally the Act breaks away from the relief-oriented programmes of the past and incorporate an integrated natural resource management and livelihoods generation perspective.

Recent official and non-official evaluations of the programme have predominantly highlighted the positive outcomes achieved by the MGNREGA. However some major problem areas have also been identified such as (*i*) limited coverage and underutilization of allocated programme funding (*ii*) slow and tardy implementation of works in some states (*iii*) the quality of works mainly due to limited technical competence of the gram panchayats in many areas and (*iv*) the significant exclusion of the old and disabled from the programme.

Suggestions for Strengthening and Improvement

Though there have been significant achievements regarding the achievement of programme objectives, there are some measures that are needed to achieve greater success and impact. These are:

Special efforts are needed to disseminate a much higher level of awareness regarding the rights based entitlements of the programme among the rural population. This is most essential for improving the penetration and coverage of the programme in many states. Additional outlays are essential for IEC and other activity to increase awareness.

There is also a need to strengthen the technical competence at the gram panchayat level by involving professional agencies and competent NGOs to train and guide panchayat members to improve the design of works that are identified for implementation. Additional outlays earmarked for this purpose should be provided.

There is an urgent need to cover the old, infirm and destitute and physically handicapped rural population by not only identifying the kind of work that they can undertake but also by increasing for them the present 100 days of assured work to at least 150 days in a year. Special job cards should be issued for this purpose.

A higher work entitlement for 150 days should also be provided to single women and women headed households.

5. CONCLUSION

In its brief introduction, this paper highlights the widely accepted definition of food security. The first section that lays out the broad contours of food security in India by providing an overview that sets the overall framework for our discussion follows this. Food Security is determined by the availability of food, the access to food and the absorption (or nutrition) of food in the system. These three conditionalities for food security are closely inter-related and thus availability and access to food can increase absorption or nutritional levels among the households.

In the second segment of the paper, an attempt has been made to analyze the broad trends and performance related to availability. It is seen that in spite of India having achieved self-sufficiency in cereals it is still lagging behind in the production of pulses and oilseeds. It is also observed that there has been a significant increase in the production of fruits, vegetables, dairy products, meat, poultry and fishery products. However per capita availability of these are still far lower than international and national norms and standards. The trends in availability appear not to be improving as required solely on account of the stagnation of the agricultural sector. An attempt has been thus made to identify the major constraints and deficiencies in agricultural growth and specific suggestions have been put forward for improving the performance of the agricultural sector and to enhance the growth rate so that it is capable of meeting the food and nutritional requirement that have been projected in the next decade. Among the specific suggestions made to lift the agricultural sector from its present slowdown and stagnation, we have highlighted increased public investment and a serious review of subsidies provided to farmers. To boost infrastructure, expansion of credit, and essential inputs, land and water management, agricultural research and extension, effective marketing and price policies, the diversification of agriculture, the strengthening of institutions catering to these needs, strengthening the mitigation strategies for tackling climate change, and the strict regulation of land use and diversion of land for non-agricultural activities.

In the next segment of this paper, focus has been shifted to the trends and performance in Access to Food and absorption/Nutrition. It is seen that there has been a perceptible decline in the levels of hunger among households; there has also been a significant lowering of the households below the poverty line. Both these trends indicate an improvement in access to food. Though there has been an improvement in urban employment the situation in rural areas is still seen to be far from satisfactory. Moreover, there has also been a noticeable increase in the number of landless labourers in the rural sector accompanied by a decline in real wages, which has affected the level of access to food in the rural as compared to the urban sector. Access to the PDS which contributes to overall access to food has generally shown an increase in practically all the regions this has been an encouraging trend, however it is also seen that the access to the PDS is still low in many states and regions.

While the performance in terms of access to food has shown an overall improvement the trends in nutrition have been far from satisfactory especially for the rural poor. The nutritional statuses particularly of children and women have not improved while the nutrition status among socially vulnerable groups of women has worsened.

An assessment of the programmes for Access to Food and Nutrition has been attempted in the final section of this paper. This section also makes a large number of suggestions for the improvement of these programmes that are intended to not only improve access to food but also to have an effective impact on the levels and status of nutrition. This part of the paper has a closer look at the TPDS, the ICDS, the MDMS as well as MGNREGA to identify the major shortcomings with these schemes and also to suggest specific measures and reforms in each of them to improve their effectiveness and impact which is most essential for ensuring food security.

The constraints in ensuring food security and reducing hunger are due to inappropriate policy, faulty design, the inadequacies in monitoring and evaluation, ineffective governance and a lack of political will. Economic growth alone is not sufficient to improve food security, reduction in malnutrition and the improvement of food intake by the poor. Without widespread reforms on various fronts and the required changes in policy coupled with an improvement in the effectiveness of implementation food security will continue to remain a daunting challenge.

Sustainable development results from efficient institutions and thus the stress on development funding must now increasingly focus on development outcomes and the effectiveness of public service delivery. The indicators of hunger among marginalized groups and of 300 million poor must be improved. This not only requires additional resources but also more effective policies and a strong delivery system.

India has designed and implemented a very wide range of programmes to enhance food security and has also succeeded to a remarkable extent however severe challenges remain on several fronts. However, the major problem is with the proper design and implementation of policies and programmes. There is in particular the urgent need to address governance issues specially those related to effective and efficient public service delivery systems. Governance needs to conform closely to the socio-economic environment and appropriate institutions are needed to improve the governance system. A people-centric and rights-based approach has shown remarkable results in the case of rural employment. It has brought about increasing transparency and accountability among those responsible for the implementation of MGNREGA.

A similar approach is being visualized for Food Security and though the National Food Security Act would burden the State and strain its exchequer it is a move in the right direction. The Act is likely to bring about a much higher level of commitment on the part of the states to meet their statutory obligations regarding food security and bringing about reform efforts on several fronts related to the food system. These reforms are necessary for India"s rapid growth and development free of social and economic instability in the years ahead.

REFERENCES

Ajani, Kumar. *et al.* (2012). „Food Security in India: Trends, Patterns, and determinants. *Indian Journal of Agricultural Economics*, Vol 67, No. 3, July-Sept 2012.

Bhalla, G.S., Hazell, P. and Kerr, J. (2001). "Prospects for India"s Cereal Supply and Demand to 2020, Food, Agriculture and the Environment, Discussion Paper 29, International Food Security Institute, Washington D.C.

Bhramanad, P.S. *et al.* (2013). "Challenges to Food Security in India". Current Science. Vol 104. No. 7, 10 April 2013.

Comptroller and Auditor General. (2007). „Performance Audit of the Implementation of National Rural Employment Guarantee Act, (20050, draft report, New Delhi.

Comptroller and Auditor General. (2008). „Performance Audit of the Implementation of the Mid Day Meal Scheme". New Delhi.

Dreze, Jean. and A. Sen. (1989). *Hunger and Public Action*, Clarendon Press. Oxford.

Dyson, Tim. and A. Hanchate. (2000). "India"s Demographic and Food Prospects: State Level Analysis", *Economic and Political Weekly*, November 11, Vol 35.

GoI. (2002). „Report of the High Level Committee on Long Term Grain Policy". Department of Food and Public Distribution System, Government of India.

GoI. (2007a). Agricultural Statistics at a Glance 2006. Directorate of Economics & Statistics, Department of Agriculture and Cooperation, Ministry of Agriculture, New Delhi.

GoI.(2007b). Report of Steering Committee on Agriculture for XIth Plan, Planning Commission, Government of India.

GoI. (2008). "Draft 11th Five year Plan". Planning Commission, Government of India.

IPCC. (2007). „Climate Change". Fourth IPCC Assessment Report, Cambridge University Press, Cambridge, United Kingdom. 2007.

Jha, Praveen. (2007). „Some Aspects of the Well Being of India"s Agricultural Labour in the Context of Contemporary Agrarian Crisis". *Indian Journal of Labour Economics, 2007.*

Jones, N., et al. (2007). „Ripple Effects or Deliberate Intentions? Assessing Linkages between Women"s Empowerment and Childhood Poverty". UNICEF/Young Lives Social Policy paper 002, May 2007.

Kumar, P. (1998). Food Demand and Supply Projections for India, Agricultural Economics Policy Paper 98-01, Division of Economics, IARI, New Delhi.

Lanjouw, P. and Rinku, M. (2009). "Poverty decline, agricultural wages and non-farm employment in rural India: 1983-2004, Policy Research Working Paper Series 4858, The World Bank.

Nema, P., Nema, S. and Roy, P. (2012). "An Overview of Global Climate Changing in Current Scenario and Mitigation Action Renewable Sustain Energy Review, Vol 16. 2012.

Patnaik, U. (2004). „The Republic of Hunger". Public lecture on the occasion of the 50th Birthday of Safdar Hashmi organized by the SAHMAT Safdar Hashmi memorial trust, New Delhi.

Planning Commission. (2005). "Performance Evaluation of the Public Distribution System". Programme Evaluation Organization, Planning Commission, Government of India.

Radhakrishna, R. and Ray, S. (2005). *Handbook of Poverty in India: Perspective, Policies and Programmes*, Oxford University Press., New Delhi.

S. Mahendra Dev and Alakh N. Sharma. (2010). Food Security in India: Performance, Challenges and Policies Oxfam India Working Paper Series, September 2010.

Saxena, N.C. (2011). Hunger, Under-Nutrition and Food Security in India. Working Paper 44, Chronic Poverty Research Centre, Indian Institute of Public Administration, New Delhi.

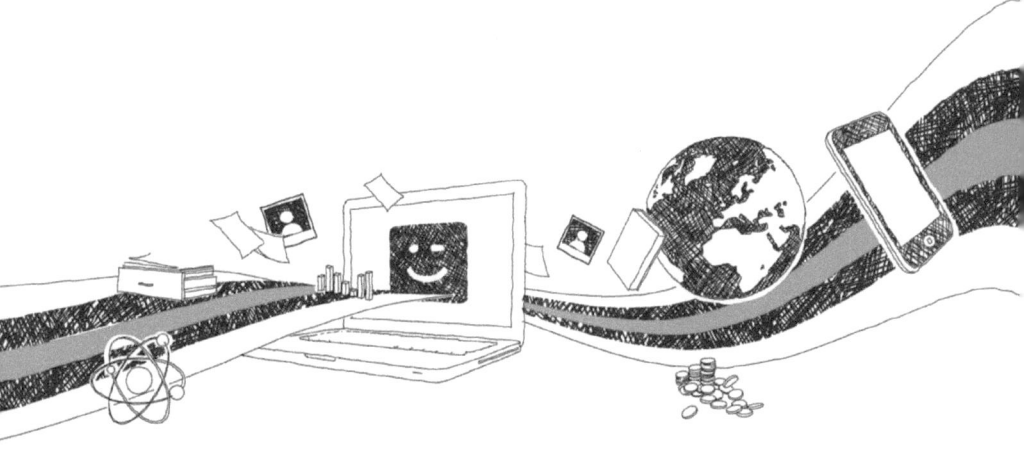
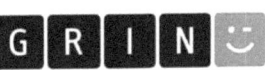